Table of Contents

Introduction

Herbal medicine is the great-great-grandmother of medicine. It is the body of medical knowledge that has been passed down from generation to generation since the early days of humanity. It is the use of simple, whole plants, complete in their natural balance of minerals, vitamins, enzymes, and active ingredients.

Developments in science and technology over the last century have enabled researchers to isolate the active ingredients from herbs, refine these ingredients into drugs, and make them conform to standard laboratory measures for what was hoped to be more predictable physical reactions. Researchers have also learned to synthesize these drugs from substances far removed from any natural source. In the process of this development, medicine, science, and technology have moved further and further away from the perfect natural balance of a simple plant. Medicine, because of its concern with disease rather than health, has moved further and further away from the human being.

The results of modern western medicine speak for themselves. Many developments of modern medicine are highly beneficial, but others create more disease than they cure. The developments in microsurgery, for instance, are so useful that I would never want to turn back the technological clock. I know, however, that many operations are not necessary if only we would stand by the simple natural balance of nature in our foods and in our medicines. My hope is that one day herbal medicine and natural medicine can work together with modern technology for the benefit of individual patients.

The human body in good working order is a natural balance of all the elements found in the earth and the plants that live on the earth. The common dandelion, for instance, has a composition of minerals, vitamins, enzymes, and active ingredients almost identical to the human liver. As a remedy, the dandelion answers the needs of every liver complaint or imbalance you can name. A number of doctors refer their hepatitis patients to me because they have seen the results of dandelion in action. After three weeks of dandelion tincture treatment (ten drops taken four times daily), my hepatitis patients are well enough to go out dancing.

It is a truth that stands to reason that the nearer we stay to the whole and natural balance of the earth and its plants, the nearer we are to our own natural balance, which we experience as health.

Herbal medicine is accessible and effective. You don't need to be a scientist to know that marigold (calendula) is antiseptic. You simply have to put it on a festering wound and watch the wound heal within twelve hours. It may be simple, but it is as effective as any and more effective than most of the chemical equivalents. You don't have to be a technician to prepare a cup of herbal tea or a poultice. Herbal medicine is the medicine of the people, and despite the sophistication of modern western medicine, it is still the preferred medicine of 90 percent of the world's population.

An herbalist today has a much wider choice of remedies than the ancient herbalists thanks to the travellers over the ages who consciously or unconsciously carried with them the seeds of their native foliage. The humble plantain is called Englishman's Foot because it sprouted wherever the English stepped. Such instances have caused ecological disasters within delicate ecosystems, but they do give herb gatherers a wide variety.

The vast distances and speed of modern travel also make available to everyone those herbs that only grow high in the Alps or in the desert. Modern herbalists have access to tinctures of plants that have never been naturalized in their own location.

No medicine chest would be large enough to house a complete herbal pharmacy. This book is a selection of a small number of herbs that most effectively treat the widest possible range of common emergencies and are readily available from health food stores, herbal pharmacies, and natural food stores in the forms described. The purpose of this book is a practical one: to fill in the gaps of information found in most popular herbals. What is the benefit of knowing that chamomile is good for the eyes if you don't know how to prepare it and how to use it?

This is not the book to use to identify the herbs in your garden or along your footpath. That sort of knowledge is best learned from someone who knows your local flora.

Herb gardeners or gatherers can, of course, make the preparations in this book from the fresh plants. However, it is dangerous to make a remedy from a plant that you cannot positively identify. It is almost impossible to identify an herb from a drawing, unless you already know the herb. If you are not sure, send the plant to the nearest university botany department or to your county extension service, where they can make a positive identification. If you are not sure, always ask someone who really does know.

A rule of thumb when gathering herbs is to stay clear of plants that have been sprayed with insecticides. No matter how much you wash the plants, the chemicals will linger and affect the remedy. These plants are not in a natural state of balance and should be avoided. Gathering should be done in wild places or where the plants are grown organically.

It is for all of these reasons I have selected herbs that are readily available commercially. Read the labels of the products you buy to see if the herbs are grown organically or picked in the wild. If this information is not on the label, write to the company and find out. All the herbs in this book are available in stores, so people who do not have the time to spend gardening or gathering can still have access to natural treatments in their own homes.

In spite of the general dissatisfaction most of us feel with chemical treatments, it takes a certain amount of courage to try Grandma's recipes in an emergency. I suggest buying a few ointments or oils at a time and trying them out as you go, until you feel confident enough with herbal treatments to throwaway the synthetic ones.

There is a general rule concerning first aid remedies, herbal or otherwise: *Keep out of the reach of children.* There are some herbs that could be dangerous if used in the wrong circumstances.

Ointments

Ointments are always used externally as dressings for skin irritations, bruises, abrasions, cuts, blisters, and the like. The benefit of using an ointment is that the base of the ointment is soothing and adds to the comfort of healing.

When buying an ointment, there are two things to look for. First, make sure the ingredients are on the label. Second, make sure the ointment is made up of at least 10 percent herbal extract. An ointment just won't do the job if it contains less than 10 percent of the herbal ingredient. The ointments mentioned in this book should all be readily available from health food stores.

Ointments should be bought or stored in brown glass jars and kept in a cool place. If a preservative is added, ointments stored in this manner will keep for several years.

HOW TO MAKE YOUR OWN OINTMENTS

Many people enjoy making their own ointments. The ingredients are readily available from health food stores, herbal pharmacies, and old-fashioned drug stores. Ointments made with herbal extracts should last as long as the ointments you buy ready-made, but those made with an herbal infusion will last only about a year.

The basic recipe for a good ointment is to combine

2 parts herbal extract
7 parts base
1 part natural preservative

You will have to buy the herbal extract. The base can be purchased or made (see below). The best natural preservative is glycerin, which is available at most drug stores.

The procedure is simple: Mix all the ingredients thoroughly. Store in a brown glass jar and keep in a cool place.

OINTMENT BASES

Raw Petroleum Jelly

Raw petroleum jelly is vegetable in origin, made from coal before it is processed. Vaseline® is petroleum jelly that has been refined three times. Using either raw or refined petroleum jelly as an ointment base requires a lot of mixing, or making the ointment in a blender it's generally a messy affair.

Lanolin

Lanolin is pure cholesterol extracted from the fleece of sheep. Although it is an animal product, it comes from the sheep's wool. It is much easier to mix and is far less messy than petroleum jelly. You must remember to use *pure* lanolin only.

Agar or Irish Moss

These are fine vegetable ointment bases. They gel nicely and have a soothing emollient action. They can be expensive, however. Here's the recipe for preparing the ointment base. The boric acid is optional; it adds an antiseptic action to the Agar.

30 grams Agar or Irish moss
300 milliliters distilled water
60 milliliters glycerin
1 teaspoon boric acid (optional)

In a large saucepan, mix the agar or Irish moss with the distilled water and bring to a gentle boil. Cover and boil gently for a few minutes. Then strain through a cheesecloth and cool. When the jelly mixture is nearly cool, mix in the glycerine and boric acid. When the mixture is completely cool, add 2 parts herbal extract to 8 parts base.

CREAMS INSTEAD OF OINTMENTS

Creams are sometimes preferred to ointments as they are absorbed more readily into the skin. In the cases of dermatitis or sunburn where large areas of skin are treated, creams are decidedly more convenient. To make a **Herbal Cream,** use any natural product skin cream, such as Vitamin E Cream, as a base and mix 2 parts herbal extract to 8 parts cream.

OINTMENTS FOR FIRSTAID

Arnica Ointment *(Arnica montana)*
Calendula or Marigold Ointment *(Calendula officinalis)*
Comfrey Ointment *(Symphytum officinale)*
Golden Seal Ointment *(Hydrastis canadensis)*
Hypericum or St. John's Wort Ointment *(Hypericum perforatum)*
Thuja Ointment *(Thuja occidentalis)*

Arnica Ointment

As its botanical name implies, Arnica grows high on the mountains just below the snow line. This member of the daisy family, with its orange-yellow flower, is native to Siberia and northern Europe. Most of the herb we use is imported.

Part Used: The flower

Uses: Treatment for bruises

Arnica is one of the best vulneraries, which means it is used for bruises. Minor or major bruises respond very quickly to Arnica Ointment. When we bruise, it is because the blood vessels beneath the skin have broken and clotted. Arnica breaks down the bruise, or blood clot, into tiny pieces. It sends the dead cells out of the tissues where the body will take over, finally sending them out through the urine.

For those times when you've smashed your thumb under a hammer and you know it will be black and blue, applying Arnica Ointment immediately will take away much of the pain and even prevent the bruise from appearing.
One warning is necessary: *Never use Arnica on broken skin or a bleeding wound.* Arnica, because it prevents blood from clotting, will make the wound bleed more. When you treat a wound that is partly bruised and partly cut, dress it with Calendula for a few days until the skin is healed, and only then treat the bruising with Arnica Ointment.

If your household has its fair share of black eyes, fingers smashed in car doors, people who ricochet off edges of furniture, or martial artists in training, you'll become aware of the importance of Arnica Ointment in the house.

Calendula or Marigold Ointment

Calendula is a hardy annual of the daisy family, well worth growing in your garden or window box. The one to grow is the common pot marigold with the golden orange flowers. The jumbos and hybrids are not medicinal.
Calendula will flower throughout the growing season if you pick the dying flowers regularly.

Part Used: The flower

Uses: As an antiseptic

Calendula is *the* household antiseptic. It is thorough and strong in its antiseptic action. Whenever you need an antiseptic, you can use Calendula in one of its many forms: ointment, poultice, or infusion. Calendula will ease any swelling, cool down the heat of inflammation, and relieve the pain of a wound. It will heal a wound from the deepest levels through to the surface damaged skin tissue, and it prevents scars' from forming.

Calendula is also a mild styptic, which means it will stop the bleeding of a wound if the bleeding is not profuse. Bloody noses stop bleeding within seconds when you put a bit of Calendula Ointment up the nose. Calendula Ointment is a first-rate treatment for all minor wounds with broken skin-from scrapes, grazes, and gravel rash to deep cuts. The best way to treat a septic or infected wound is to wash it with Calendula Infusion (see Teas and Infusions), then dress it with Calendula Ointment or a simple Calendula poultice.

To make a simple poultice, thoroughly bruise a marigold flower in a mortar and pestle and dress the wound with it. Only use flowers that have been grown organically. Putting commercial sprays on a septic wound is *not* a good idea. Insecticides are a very good reason *not* to gather the flowers from public parks.

Comfrey Ointment

Comfrey, a member of the borage family, is native to Europe and temperate Asia and will grow anywhere. Even under the worst conditions, Comfrey will thrive; it fed the

Irish during the potato famine. Once you have Comfrey in your garden, you'll have it forever! Its leaves are large, green, and hairy. The bottom leaves grow as large as ten to sixteen inches long. It is propagated by root division in autumn.

Parts Used: The leaf and root

Uses: To prevent and treat scar tissue and promote rapid healing

Comfrey leaf and Comfrey root are occasionally used in different circumstances. The leaf contains more enzymes than the root and is best used on festering wounds, such as skin ulcers and bedsores, where putrid tissue must be cleaned up. In my experience, the best skin ulcer treatment is an ointment mixture of Calendula, Comfrey leaf, and Comfrey root. Comfrey root is rich in vitamin B-12 and contains a cell proliferant.

The most convenient ointment to have in the medicine chest is the brown Comfrey Ointment, which is a mixture of leaf and root.

Burns and Blisters

Comfrey Ointment is the basic herbal treatment for all sorts of burns, from minor burns and blistered sunburns to third-degree burns. When we burn ourselves, we break or destroy the cell walls, and the plasma, containing the basic cell nutrients, leaks out of the cells to form a blister. Unless the blister breaks, a burn is considered a sterile wound, so there is no need to use an antiseptic.
Comfrey seals the wound and heals the burn so quickly that if you dress a burn immediately with Comfrey Ointment,

the blister you would have expected does not even appear. Comfrey also takes the pain and
the heat away very quickly.

The very first thing to do with any burn is to cool it to prevent the burn from reaching deeper into the tissue. Soak the affected area in ice water for several minutes.

Then seal it by dressing with Comfrey Ointment. With severe burns, change the dressing twice daily until any mark of the burn is gone. Comfrey leaves no scars.

Scar Prevention

Comfrey root prevents scarring by its cell proliferant action. Comfrey root contains allantoin, which is found in the urine of pregnant women and babies. Its presence is an indication that the cells are dividing and reproducing quickly and normally. Allantoin grows normal healthy cells at 3 times the standard rate and replaces dead cells at the same speed. Comfrey root also contains vitamin B-12, the master vitamin, which controls the cell replacement rate and insures that only normal and healthy cells are being reproduced. Comfrey is a cell normaliser, as well as a cell proliferant, eating up the dead cells with its enzyme action and replacing them with normal cells at a very fast rate. It is this action that prevents scar tissue from forming. Any wound that you think might leave a scar will not do so if you continue to dress it with Comfrey Ointment until it is thoroughly healed.

It is safe to use Comfrey Ointment on postoperative scars only if there is no risk of infection. As Comfrey is not an antiseptic, it is best to dress postoperative wounds with Calendula, until you are sure they are free of infection. Then switch to Comfrey Ointment dressings.

Old Scars

Whether it is pock marks left over from teenage acne,
stretch marks from the last pregnancy, the old appendix
scar, or even those premature wrinkles, all will respond to
Comfrey root. Comfrey Root Cream is the most convenient
treatment. Massage it into the scarred area nightly.

A more intensive treatment is Dorothy Hall's recipe for
Comfrey Root Goo: Put a handful of fresh Comfrey root in
a saucepan with water to cover. Bring it to a boil and then
simmer. Slowly a cream will form. Mash the root as best
you can after it has cooked for a while. When the "goo" has
formed, strain out any bits of root. Use the Comfrey Root
Goo as an overnight mask, washing it off the next morning.
Do this twice a week and the scars or wrinkles will
disappear. The older the scar, the longer the treatment is
necessary, but you will be able to see the changes.

Skin Irritations

Allergic reactions, rough hands from too harsh a
dishwashing liquid, itching eczema, and diaper rash are all
soothed with Comfrey Cream. It is not always a complete
treatment, but it is soothing and heals any breaks in the
skin.

Cuts and Abrasions

The one thing to remember about Comfrey is that it is not
an antiseptic. If you treat an infected cut with Comfrey it
can heal too fast, actually sealing the infection in, and you
will have to draw it out later. It is best to use Calendula first
if there are any worries of infection. If you are treating a

clean cut, it is safe to use Comfrey Ointment immediately. It will heal rapidly and scarlessly.

Golden Seal Ointment

Golden Seal, a member of the buttercup family, grows best in its native North America, in the rich soil of shady woods. It is a small perennial herb with a horizontal, golden yellow rootstock. Golden Seal is one of the most healing of herbs, and, unfortunately, one of the most expensive, due to over collection and urban expansion.

Part Used: The root

Uses: Skin softening and normalizing

Used as an ointment, Golden Seal has a softening, soothing, and normalizing action on callused skin, corns, and bunions. Any corroded skin condition, such as pock marks, or any chronic peeling skin also responds to the soothing and normalizing action of Golden Seal.

Massage the ointment thoroughly into the hardened or corroded area until it is completely absorbed. You can see the skin soften and stop peeling within a matter of days.

As Golden Seal is also a dye, any excess ointment will stain your clothes or bedclothes.

Hypericum Ointment

Hypericum Ointment is made from St. Johns's Wort, a common pasture weed found in uncultivated open meadows and by roadsides. Growing up to 3 feet tall, this shrub by herb has bright yellow flowers.

Part Used: The flowers

Uses: Treatment for nerve ending damage or irritation Hypericum Ointment calms down any overreaction of the nerve endings in the skin.

It is good for hypersensitive allergic skin reactions, stings of insects, or nettle rashes. It soothes the sharp stinging needle pains by calming and normalizing the nerve endings. After any major skin damage, as with burns, accidents, or operations, healing can be a painful experience. When the numbness leaves and the nerve endings begin to heal, we feel a severe pins-and-needles pain.

Using Hypericum Ointment as a dressing while the skin is still numb will restore the sense of feeling and prevent the acute nerve ending pain during the healing process. I have also known Hypericum Ointment to mend severed nerve endings and ease the ghost pains that people suffer after a limb has been amputated. If your household runs on the do-it-yourself concept, Hypericum Ointment is definitely one to have on hand. Many a finger chopped off by a power saw and many great chunks of flesh that have met the mincer have regained their function thanks to Hypericum.

Oils

Oils for First Aid

In the case of a major infection of the chest or abdominal regions, when you can feel congestion in the glands and tissues, it is wise to get rid of the infected matter as quickly as possible. This is most quickly done using a combination of internal treatments, such as garlic or slippery elm, which will break up the congestion and send it out of the body through the eliminatory organs; and external drawing treatments, such as a Castor Oil Pack, which will break up the congestion and draw it our through the skin.

Castor Oil Pack

To make a Castor Oil Pack, you will need an old towel large enough to wrap around the torso and be secured at the back with a safety pin. You will also need a plastic bag large enough to cover the infected area. Small garbage bags are excellent for this purpose. Lastly, you will need a double thickness of an old sheet, the same size as the plastic bag.

Castor Oil has drawing power up to 4 inches deep, and it draws thoroughly. All bits of rust or any other nasties are drawn out, preventing all kinds of infection. Pour the Castor Oil onto a wad of cotton wool, where it will sit in a small puddle. Apply it to the wound and wrap it up. Change the dressing every two hours for the rest of the day, and twice daily for the next three days. You can safely forget about tetanus or any other kind of infection. Castor Oil will draw abscesses. It will draw out the irritation of tick bites, as well as any tick heads that were left behind in the tug-of-war. It will draw out splinters, and it will draw out infection from any part of the body you can put a poultice or pack on.

Lay the towel on a flat surface. Place the plastic bag in the middle of the towel and place the double sheeting on top of the plastic. Now you need to warm the Castor Oil. Put the bottle in a pan of hot water and let it stand for about 5 minutes. The oil should pour easily when it is warm. Pour the warm Castor Oil all over the top piece of double-layer sheeting, spreading it as evenly as possible.

Place the entire pack, the oil side directly on the skin, to cover the infected area. Wrap the outer towel around the body and pin it securely in place. The pack should be kept in place overnight for three nights in a row. The drawing action of Castor Oil is quite visible. When you remove the pack in the morning, the inner sheeting will be discoloured with the infected matter that has been drawn out.

Never recycle the inner sheeting.

Throw it away.

Eyes

The drawing action of Castor Oil is very useful with the rather serious emergency of having a splinter in the eye, or any matter deeply buried in the eye tissue that does not respond to the Golden Seal eye wash (see Golden Seal Extract). The thick oiliness of Castor Oil oozes the splinter, or foreign matter, out slowly and will not tear or damage the sensitive eye tissue.

For splinters in the eye, metal or otherwise, put 3 drops of Castor Oil directly into the eye, place an eye pad of cotton wool soaked in Calendula Infusion (see Teas and Infusions) over the eyelid, wrapping it up for 12 hours. It does sting the eye initially, but it is a soothing treatment and the splinter should appear on the surface of the eye ready to be carefully picked up. If it is not, repeat the treatment. When the splinter has been removed, pack the closed eye with cotton wool soaked in Castor Oil and wrap it up for another 12 hours. This is to insure that the eye is free of infection.

Serious Eye Infections

Any eye infection that does not rapidly respond to the cleansing Golden Seal eye wash (see Golden Seal Extract) will certainly respond to Castor Oil. Pack the closed eye with cotton wool soaked in Castor Oil and wrap it up. Eye masks are perfect for keeping an eye pack in place. The relief is almost immediate, but keep the eye pack on overnight. In the morning when you remove the pack, you will not be able to open your eyes because they will be gummed up with matter drawn by the Castor Oil. Wash the eyes with either Golden Seal wash (see Golden Seal Extract) or Calendula Infusion (see Teas and Infusions). Repeat this overnight treatment until you can freely open your eyes in the morning.

Eucalyptus Oil

Eucalyptus Oil comes mostly from the blue gum tree, but many other species also have a high oil content in their fresh leaves, and all species are medicinal.

Uses: Antiseptic and expectorant

Eucalyptus is the most powerfully antiseptic of the oils, and it grows more strongly antiseptic when it is old. A substance called ozone is formed in the bottle once the oil is exposed to air, and this aids the disinfectant action. Eucalyptus works primarily in the respiratory system.

Inhalant

One way to relieve all congestion of a cold or flu from the sinuses to the chest is to inhale Eucalyptus. Boil some water, turn off the heat, and put a few drops of Eucalyptus Oil in it. You could also use mashed fresh leaves and new shoots instead of the oil. With your head over the pot of water, drape a towel to make a tent over your head and the water and inhale. Never inhale over boiling water. Using Eucalyptus as an inhalant gets to the heart of the infection because of its antiseptic action. It is also useful for laryngitis and other throat problems as well as dry sinuses or aching raw sinuses.

Chest Rub

As a chest rub, Eucalyptus Oil has a very penetrating action, opening up the air passages and fighting infection. If your skin is at all sensitive, it may be best to dilute Eucalyptus Oil with a bland healing oil, such as wheat germ oil, before applying it to the chest.

Internally

For severe bronchial or lung infections you can use Eucalyptus Oil internally, but watch the dose. Small doses are all you need and large doses are dangerous, so don't overdo it. For chronic chest conditions or for a cold that has been hanging around for months, taking 2 drops of Eucalyptus Oil in 1 teaspoon of honey once a day for a week will shake it. Eucalyptus has been used internally to treat tuberculosis and other microbe lung diseases quite successfully in European TB sanatoriums, where it was found that Eucalyptus Oil actually kills the TB organism outright.

Bath Oil

Putting a few drops of Eucalyptus Oil in the bath stimulates the circulation and relaxes the muscular aches and pains that often accompany a cold or flu. It also has the effect of taking a bath in an inhaler. A Eucalyptus Oil bath is a complete and relaxing cold and flu treatment.

Eucalyptus Oil baths also work wonders for muscular aches and pains after too strenuous a workout. When you have proved to yourself that you are as fit as ever and played your first game of squash in five years, a good soak in a Eucalyptus Oil bath will mean no stiff muscles the next day. It's a good treatment for the ego as well as the muscles.
I.
Skin Parasites

For any skin parasites, such as ringworm or scabies, soak a cloth in Eucalyptus Oil and rub it on the infected area twice daily until it is gone. If the skin is too sensitive, it may be better to make a strong infusion of the leaves for this purpose (see Teas and Infusions).

Stain Remover

Here is one household use we could not possibly overlook. All sorts of stains on clothing come out when you dab a bit of Eucalyptus Oil on them. The sooner you treat a stain, the easier it will be to remove. Even with old stains, however, if you soak a bit of cotton wool in Eucalyptus Oil and rub it on the stain, letting it dry before you wash it, it usually comes clean.

Lavender is native to the mountainous Mediterranean regions and spread with the Romans wherever they travelled. Today it is a common garden plant. If you want your picked Lavender to last with its distinctive aroma, harvest it in full flower as midsummer approaches. The oil will then be concentrated in the flower.

Uses: Toning and calming the nerves

Headaches

Lavender Oil is good for a specific type of headache that starts with tension at the neck and base of the skull. It is the sort of headache that can be the cause of insomnia no matter how you rest your head on the pillow, it will not relax. Lavender Oil rubbed on the back of the neck and worked into the base of the skull will ease all the tension very quickly. It is also a good idea to brush your hair thoroughly from the underside to draw out some of the tension you have accumulated in your head. You should sleep relaxed and wake refreshed and ready to go, even after a short nap.

Natural Sedative

Lavender Oil acts as a natural sedative with no side effects or hangovers. In circumstances of shock, panic, hysteria, and for a feeling of faintness with shock or sunstrokes, simply hold the bottle of Lavender Oil under the nose and rub a bit of it on the back of the neck. In cases of emergencies, it works very quickly, restoring calm within minutes.

Linseed Oil comes from the common flax plant that grows the world over and has done so for so many centuries that its native land is unknown. We get linen from the stems and oil from the seed. Linseed Oil is best bought from a health food store.

Uses: Massage for ligaments

Linseed Oil used as massage oil is perfect treatment for strained, sprained, stretched, twisted, and torn ligaments. It works just as well for the tight ligaments as it does for the loose ones because it tones the ligaments as well as restores their elasticity.

Linseed Oil is as essential in sports medicine as it is in home first aid for the sprained ankles and twisted knees that are an inherent part of the human experience. Massage the sprained area every few hours when the pain is acute, and follow up with a daily massage of the area until the joint has totally recovered.

Olive Oil comes from the olive. The olive tree is native to Asia Minor and is cultivated in most warm climates. For first aid, it is best to buy a small bottle of the virgin oil, which comes from the first pressing of the olive.

Uses: Lubrication and calming of sensitive skin and ears
Olive Oil plays an important role in the diet, with its prevention of gallstone patterns and its strong lubricating ability.

Most dry skin and dry scalp conditions improve with the simple addition of more oil to the diet. Olive Oil also contains natural sodium chloride, which gets the gastric juices working and insures a good appetite as well as better digestion.

Ears

Olive Oil is the basic ingredient of herbal ear drops, which are useful for treating ears that tend to waxy build-ups, ears that discharge, ears that catch cold winds, or ears that ache. If there is an infection deep in the ear, you can mix a bit of Castor Oil with the Olive Oil to add to its drawing power.

Warm up a bit of Olive Oil by putting a small jar of it in a bowl of warm water. Put 3 drops in each ear and rub in the ear. Leave it overnight and clean the ears with a bit of cotton wool the next morning. It gives pain relief and a good general cleaning of the ears.

Skin Rashes

In all cases of skin rash, and allergic rash in particular, Olive Oil rubbed on the affected area will calm down the reaction with its soothing action. Olive Oil is bland, soothing, and lubricating to the skin and scalp, which is why it is one of the ingredients in so many good quality soaps and shampoos.

Dry Scalp

For dry scalp dandruff, Grandma's old Olive Oil treatment is one of the best. Warm some Olive Oil, adding any scent you like, and massage it well into the scalp. Keep it on as long as you can before washing it out. Wrap your head in a towel if it is a cool day or, if you want to bring out the highlights in your hair, sit in the sun.

Rosemary, the shrub that gives us our kitchen herb, is native to the Mediterranean and will grow wherever the sun shines. It prefers sandy and rocky soil.

Uses: Toning and relaxing nerves and muscles

Tension Headaches

Rosemary is treatment for the tension headache, that throbbing in the temples that usually comes with the gritting of teeth or the squinting and straining of eyes. Massage a bit of Rosemary Oil on the temples and across the forehead. If you clench your jaw when you are tense, lightly massage Rosemary Oil along your jaw line as well. The nerves of the face will relax smartly and the headache will ease.

If tension headaches are a fact of your lifestyle, you should see how you can change your lifestyle to make it less stressful. Remember, pain is a barometer of health.

Muscles

Tight muscles, muscles in spasm, painfully strained muscles, or those weak, floppy, untoned muscles all respond to a massage of Rosemary Oil. Rosemary Oil will tone up and relax the muscles, which is why it is often an ingredient of massage oils. If your household is on the sporting side, you may want to make up a mixture of half-and-half Rosemary and Linseed Oils. With this combination oil on your shelf, you will be ready to treat strained muscles and strained ligaments in the same massage.

Hair Conditioner

If you have dark hair, Rosemary will keep your hair healthy, shiny, and dark. After you have washed your hair, put a few drops of Rosemary Oil on your hair brush and brush it through. It won't make your hair greasy. It will keep your hair looking and smelling nice. You can get a similar effect by using Rosemary Infusion for the final rinse after shampooing your hair (see Teas and Infusions).

Sandalwood Oil

Sandalwood Oil comes from the wood of the sandalwood tree. It is native to India and has straw-colored flowers that turn deep reddish purple when they open.

Uses: Protection of the aura

Sandalwood is a necessity for sensitive, intuitive, and 'psychic' types of people. It is for the people who listen to other people's problems-the counsellors, the healers, and the neighbourhood ear to whom everyone comes for guidance and nurturing. You know when you need it. It is for the times when, though you were feeling fresh and alive before your friend or client came, they left you suffering with the headache they complained of, their rheumatic pains, or their heart-breaking sadness. They feel much better, of course, and are bound to call again, so you had better be ready for the next visit!

It may be because of love or compassion for these people that you actually take their sadness or pain inside yourself in order to make them feel better. You are blending their life force, or aura, with your own. Our aura, or electrical force field, is our first line of defence.

It acts very much like a permeable membrane, filtering out certain influences that may be harmful, yet allowing un-harmful influences in. It can become a big problem if, because of compassion, someone has left their aura wide open. The greater problem arises when compassionate, intuitive persons think they are going around the bend because they are suffering one set of symptoms or another each time they have a visitor.

There is a solution: Sandalwood Oil, of course! Put a drop of Sandalwood Oil on your third eye, in the middle of your brow just above your nose. Put another drop on the seventh cervical vertebra (C7) of your neck. You will find the vertebra is prominent in the neck when you hang your head forward. You should be able to feel that vertebra just above your shoulder line. Within minutes after using Sandalwood Oil in this way, you will find the aches, pains, and sadness you picked up from your friend or client begins to fade. Sandalwood Oil is sealing your aura, if you believe in that sort of thing. Using Sandalwood Oil as a preventative can enhance or even develop your psychic ability, intuition, or compassion, because you won't feel drained every time you listen to someone's problems. Some people need to use Sandalwood Oil daily.

Teas and Infusions

Herbs are used as medicines in the home primarily in the form of teas and infusions. They are the nutritional part of herbal medicine, used to supplement the diet and ease the side effects of bad habits.

When you need to relieve pains or acute symptoms of ill health, drinking a cup of herbal tea or a glass of infusion will certainly help. Infusions generally are used when the symptoms are more acute because the infusions are twice as strong as teas. The beauty of herbal teas, however, is in preventing illness. It takes time to correct a pattern of ill health, so taking the right herbal tea as a regular part of your diet will prevent the illness, and therefore the symptoms, from recurring.

Teas and infusions can also be used externally as a wash for any part of the body. Simply let the tea or infusion cool down so that it can be applied externally. They can also be used as a final rinse after washing your hair. One or two cups of a tea or infusion can be added to the bath for a total body treatment. Dressings for wounds or sprains can be prepared by soaking the dressing in the tea or infusion and applying it to the affected area. Strong infusions can be used in making creams and ointments. Teas and infusions are made easily in the kitchen using either dried herbs or herbs fresh from the garden.

Dried herbs can last for several years if they are properly dried and stored in airtight containers. You can buy dried herbs in supermarkets, health food stores, herbal pharmacies, and by the mail. A packet of 3 ½ ounces of a dried herb is a good amount to buy when you are starting out. It will give you a chance to find out which herbs you use more frequently before you buy in bulk. Some of the more popular herbal teas are available in tea bags, making it very convenient if you want only one cup. When using fresh herbs, it is best to bruise the herb with a mortar and pestle before adding it to the teapot.

MAKING AN HERBAL TEA

Making an herbal tea is much the same as making black tea. Use 1 teaspoon of dried herb for each person and 1 for the pot. Fresh herbs are, of course, harder to measure because of varying sizes of leaf and sprig. A small handful of the fresh herb will generally make a nice cup of tea. Add boiling water, let it steep a few minutes (the longer the steeping, the stronger the brew), strain with an ordinary tea strainer, and drink. You generally do not add milk to herbal tea, though adding a spoon of honey will make it very palatable.

MAKING AN INFUSION

Making an infusion is much the same as making a strong tea. Use about 1 ounce of dried herb, or 4 small handfuls of fresh herb, to a small, 3-cup teapot. Pour boiling water over the herb, let it steep until it is cool, and strain with an ordinary tea strainer. Infusions will keep in the refrigerator for a few days. A standard dose of infusion for internal uses is a full wine glass 3 times daily.

Never use aluminum teapots for herbal teas. Porcelain or pottery teapots are best, as the herb will not be affected by the clay. This applies mainly to the brewing stage of preparation and does not necessarily apply to the tea strainer. Some people use a special teapot for herbal teas because the flavour of black tea is changed when made in the same pot. It is a matter of taste.

DRIED HERBS FORTEAS AND INFUSIONS FOR FIRST AID

Calendula *(Calendula officinalis)*
Coltsfoot *(Iussilago farfara)*
Chamomile *(Matricaria chamomilla; Antbemis nobilis)*
Rosehip *(Rosa canine)*
Senna *(Cassia acutijolia)*

Calendula Tea & Infusion

Calendula, the household antiseptic, is worth using as an infusion any time you need an antiseptic wash.

Part Used: The flowers

Uses: Antiseptic

For cleaning up a wound or as a facial wash for infected skin conditions, such as acne, Calendula Infusions work wonders. You can also dress a wound by soaking the dressing in a strong infusion.

Swellings

Swellings of all sorts calm down when washed or dressed with Calendula Infusion. It is lovely as a footbath for infected or swollen feet. To make a proper footbath, add a quart of boiling water to a handful of Calendula flowers and when it is cool enough, soak you feet.

Eyes

Calendula has a special affinity for the eyes. For infected eyes, conjunctivitis, inflamed eyes, sties, or tired eyes, use a cool Calendula Infusion as an eye wash. If it is an acute eye condition, wash the eyes 3 or 4 times daily. If it is not, washing the eyes morning and night will fight any infection, ease inflammation, and refresh them. If you are going to take a nap, make some Calendula eye pads by soaking some cotton wool in Calendula Infusion.

Place them on your eyes during your nap. When you awake, your eye will sparkle and your vision will be very clear.

Vaginal Douche

With any bacterial type of vaginal or genital infection and irritation, using Calendula Infusion as a douche, or even patting it on the genitals, will calm down the itch, heat, and inflammation. It will generally bring comfort. In some instances of genital inflammation, it is a complete treatment. If you have a chronic problem with vaginal infections, see your herbalist-stronger treatments may be necessary.

Mild Depression

Whenever you are down in the dumps and feel like singin' the blues, Calendula Tea does a good deal to lift the spirits and warm the heart.

Coltsfoot Tea & Infusion

Coltsfoot is a member of the daisy family and is native to Europe, North Africa, and Asia. In North America, it is one of the earliest spring flowers, resembling dandelions in colour and form. Its hoof-shaped leaves, covered in fine downy hairs, have given Coltsfoot its country name.

Parts Used: The root and leaves, and occasionally the flowers

Uses: Expectorant

Coughs and Chest Conditions

Coltsfoot is an expectorant. It removes mucus and phlegm from the pleural cavity, lungs, and bronchial tree. It eases wheezing and shortness of breath by opening the air passages and toning the nerve supply to the chest area. This also has the effect of easing any spasmodic coughing. If someone in your home is prone to chest conditions or asthma, Coltsfoot Tea as a common beverage is first-rate preventative medicine.

As an infusion, Coltsfoot is a stronger treatment and useful for bronchitis, flu, pneumonia, and even whooping cough and asthma. Coltsfoot is very useful to the frail or the aged when a cough sets in. The expectorant action of Coltsfoot helps to get behind the mucus and almost does the coughing for you, leaving you less exhausted.

In more severe chest conditions, such as emphysema, pleurisy, pneumonia, whooping cough, and asthma, you will need stronger doses of Colts foot and other herbs, so it is best to see an herbalist. In the meantime, Coltsfoot Infusion taken 3 times a day will bring comfort.

Chamomile Tea

Chamomile, one of the favourites of the herb garden, is very useful in first aid. Both the creeping variety *(Anthemis nobilis)* and the taller variety *(Matricaria cbamomilia)* are medicinal, though the latter is stronger.

Part Used: The flowers

Uses: Digestive tonic and soporific

Digestion

Poor digestion is probably the most common complaint of the western world. **It** is likely that someone in your home could benefit by drinking Chamomile Tea. Chamomile Tea neutralizes excess stomach acid. **It** both prevents and treats indigestion. It tones underactive stomachs, insuring complete digestion. It calms stomach aches, spasm, and tension; dispels nausea; releases painful, trapped wind and colic; and soothes stomach ulcers. Drinking Chamomile Tea regularly will change your digestive patterns.

Tension Eating

When you grab a bit to eat on the run in between your frantic chores, have too many working lunches, or nibble away at the cookies whenever you are tense or depressed, you will have a hard time digesting your food.

If your stomach is in a knot, it is hardly likely to work properly. Those few extra inches around the waistline often result from this simple problem. If this is your usual eating pattern, drinking Chamomile Tea regularly will insure proper digestion by relaxing your stomach and making the best of the food you've eaten. If you suffer too many stomach complaints, please look at your eating patterns.

Overeating and Anorexia

Overeating often comes down to tension eating, whether it's eating while you are tense or using food to swallow down those emotions that are about to erupt but are too painful to experience. Some people overeat to satisfy a hunger that food cannot fill, like a hunger for company or for love. They eat and eat and eat and never feel satisfied. They have lost the hunger reflex.

Anorexia is the refusal to eat. Anorexia and overeating are opposite sides of the same coin. Some people refuse nourishment for emotional reasons, and others eat to fill the emotional emptiness. Effective treatment lies in the emotional sphere. Confronting your feelings is the cure. Chamomile Tea will, however, calm down that overworked stomach. It will digest the food of the overeater and neutralize the intense acidity of the anorexic.

Headaches

Chamomile Tea is correct treatment for sick headaches where your stomach and head are both swimming. This headache usually starts with swallowing (gulp) tension, and the ache then bounces from the stomach to the head. Many migraine patterns have their beginning stages in this type of headache. Chamomile Tea for a youngster with sick headaches could prevent a life of migraines.

Sleep

Chamomile Tea is the perfect evening drink if you have a problem getting to sleep or waking in the night. Chamomile is a soporific and lulls you to a restful sleep. Certain types of insomnia are linked to indigestion. In these instances,

Chamomile Tea in the evenings is just about complete treatment.

Menstrual Pain

Drinking a cup of Chamomile Tea alleviates menstrual spasms.

Babies and Toddlers

Chamomile is one of baby's best all-around remedies. As well as preventing and treating bowel and stomach pains, colic, and diarrhoea, it has a number of other uses.

The daily bottle of Chamomile Tea with a bit of honey (the honey increases the calcium absorption rate) gives the baby calcium phosphate for growing healthy bones and teeth, minimizes the trauma of teething by calming the pain and nausea, and helps the baby to sleep soundly. For the pain of teething, you can also put a small handful of Chamomile flowers in a handkerchief, warm it on a hot kettle, and hold it to the jaw.

Internally, and externally as a wash, Chamomile Tea does wonders for all sorts of infant skin rashes and cradle cap. It is also a lovely eye wash for gummed-up eyes.

Pregnancy

During pregnancy, Chamomile is one of the herbs that insures enough calcium phosphate for Mom's hair, teeth, and nails, as well as the baby's growing bones. It will also ease morning sickness.

Rosehip Tea & Infusion

Rosehip comes from the pink wild rose that grows on land that has been tilled then left to grow wild. It is common in temperate regions the world over.
Uses: Circulatory tonic; complete source of vitamin C If you have any circulatory problems, from varicose veins to a heart condition, Rosehip Tea should be one of your regular beverages. It is a safe circulatory tonic in all circumstances.

With its combination of vitamin C and its action as a circulatory tonic, Rosehip is the perfect drink for times of too much physical stress or anxiety. Whenever you feel that you just cannot cope or that you are falling to pieces, Rosehip Tea is a safe and sure pick-me-up.

It will give you the energy to deal with your situation effectively.

Resistance to Infection

If you are run down, or have been living on adrenalin for too many days in a row, your resistance to any infection will be low. Rosehip Tea taken whenever you feel run down will restore your natural resistance and help prevent colds and flu.

If you already have a cold, flu, or any infection, have a teacup of Rosehip Infusion 3 times daily. It will help localize infection as well as help you to fight it.

Adults: 6-10 pods
Children: 3-5 pods
Infants: 2 pods

Drink a teacup of the infusion at night after a few hours without food, and the bowels will move in the morning. They will return to their normal pattern the next day.

If you are mildly constipated as a general pattern, you can use the Senna Pod Infusion regularly, with no side effects except improvement in the tone of your bowel. If you suffer a severe constipation pattern and have come to rely on a laxative to make your bowels move at all, see your herbalist. Stronger herbal treatment will be necessary as your bowels have forgotten how to work on their own.

Tinctures and Extracts

Tinctures and extracts are the strongest forms of herbal medicine. In these forms, the essence of the herb is concentrated in an alcohol base. Most herbs give their characters and qualities to alcohol more efficiently than they do to water, and because alcohol is so rapidly absorbed into the bloodstream, herbs taken in a tincture or extract form are fast-acting and even dramatic in their effect. An added benefit of the alcohol base is the extended shelf life it affords. Extracts will last up to 7 years, and tinctures up to 10 years; and they will still be as effective as when they were first made-provided they are kept in brown bottles and in a cool place.

The major difference between tinctures and extracts is in their effect. Tinctures are a more vibrational treatment and will affect the whole person. Herbalists skilled at dosages can treat imbalances on mental, emotional, and spiritual levels, as well as the physical level, using tinctures. Extracts, on the other hand, have a very strong physical effect; and depending on the herb, extracts can sometimes be too strong to be taken internally.

For home use, it is a general rule to use tinctures internally, taken in a mouth full of water, and to use extracts externally in the form of washes, creams, and ointments.

All tinctures and extracts used in a medicinal practice must, by law, conform to laboratory measures. Beginning herbalists may find it far more convenient and safer to buy the tinctures and extracts for first aid.

For household use, l-ounce bottles of the tinctures and extracts listed below will probably keep you in stock for a year. They are available from herbal pharmacies and health food stores, and through the mail.

TINCTURES AND EXTRACTS FOR FIRST AID

Black Cohosh Tincture *(Cimicifuga racemosa)*
Golden Seal Extract *(Hydrastis canadensis)*
Yarrow Tincture *(Achillea millefolium)*

Black Cohosh Tincture

A member of the ranuncula family, Black Cohosh, with its white candle-like flowers, is native to eastern North America. When you put this little bottle on the shelf of your medicine chest, label it "Emergency Only."

Part Used: The root

Uses: For severe and observable spasms

Black Cohosh is a very powerful antispasmodic. All types of fits and convulsions respond to Black Cohosh, as do the severe spasms of croup and whooping cough.

You can use Black Cohosh with certain menstrual cramps, but only for the violent uterine cramps complete with migraine and nausea.

Black Cohosh doesn't remedy the cause of the spasm, it simply relaxes it. It is used only while there is spasm and will cause a spasm if there is none for it to counteract.

For these reasons it is a 1-dose or 2-dose treatment. Put 7 drops of Black Cohosh Tincture directly on the tongue each 15 minutes. For children, use 4 drops each 15 minutes. It will be absorbed immediately. If someone's jaw is locked during a fit, either rub the tincture on the lips or on the pulse.

Croup and Whooping Cough

It is safe to use Black Cohosh each time there is an attack of spasmodic coughing. There is an added bonus in that Black Cohosh also has an expectorant action and will help you to cough up anything that should be coughed up. You will need other herbs to complete the treatment, so it is best to see an herbalist in these situations.

Birthing

Many a midwife in the practice of natural childbirth will know the benefit of Black Cohosh during labour. Seven drops of Black Cohosh every hour during labour will ease the spasms, relax the woman, and shorten labour. For this specific use, one of the country names for Black Cohosh is Squaw Root.

Golden Seal Extract

Golden Seal Extract is useful in first aid for some of its external uses. Golden Seal is rich in vitamin A.

Uses: For the eyes and mucus membrane

Eyes

With minor eye complaints, such as conjunctivitis, sties, tired red eyes, or the scratchy, sandy feeling of a foreign particle in the eye, a Golden Seal bath brings immediate relief that lasts all day. It has an antiseptic and cleansing action for any infection, a drawing power to clean out any foreign particle, and soothing resins to calm any irritation.

For serious eye conditions, Golden Seal has a deep action in the eyeball and will get well into the structure and fluid of the eye with its soothing detergent and antiseptic action. It is an important part of herbal treatment in serious eye conditions, such as glaucoma, but it is not complete.

To make an eye wash, put 2 drops of Golden Seal Extract into an eye cup of warm water and bathe the eyes morning and night.

Genital Infections

Whenever there is genital inflammation, pain, or irritation due to any cause, Golden Seal will soothe it. Make a mixture of 15 drops of Golden Seal Extract to a cup of warm water and pat it on the genitals or use it as a douche. The irritation and pain of vaginitis, herpes, and even STDs will respond to Golden Seal.

With most forms of vaginitis, the combination of Golden Seal as a douche and a course of Garlic Oil Capsules is complete treatment. In cases of major sexual infections, see a practitioner immediately. The major problem of genital infections is reinfection, and both parties need to be treated.

Yarrow Tincture

Yarrow, with its white to mauve flowers and feathery leaves, is a member of the daisy family. It is a common plant in herb gardens and is known as the plant's physician as it helps liven up any ailing plants around it.

Part Used: The whole plant

Uses: Astringent and styptic

Haemorrhage

In its tincture form, Yarrow will stop a haemorrhage, from a bleeding ulcer to a major haemorrhage from any organ. Even in cases of haemophilia, Yarrow will stop the bleeding.

Whenever there is a profuse, steady flow of blood, take 10 drops of Yarrow Tincture on the tongue each 10 minutes until the bleeding stops. A few doses is all that is usually necessary. Yarrow is not a complete treatment, but it is very useful while you are waiting for an ambulance. Yarrow also helps to boost the vitality that is usually fading fast in times of haemorrhage and severe fluid loss.

Fluid Loss

In cases of severe fluid loss, as with dysentery or prolonged diarrhoea where there are fears of dehydration, take 10 drops (5 drops for children) of Yarrow Tincture in a bit of water every few hours until the pattern eases. Again, it is not complete treatment, though it will calm the symptoms and boost the vitality.

Garlic Oil Capsules

Garlic Oil comes from the common garlic *(Allium sativznn)* found in most kitchens. Those who regularly cook with garlic will not need medicinal doses as frequently as those who do not.

The benefit of capsules is, of course, their convenience. It is more convenient and less socially dangerous in some circles, to take capsules rather man to chew a clove or two. It is remarkable, though, how many children will chew the capsules. Children are generally more instinctual in their eating man adults, and often less concerned with social standards. With these children, 2 cloves of crushed garlic on a slice of bread and butter will give the same results as 6 garlic capsules.
You can prepare a garlic honey for medicinal use.

Thoroughly crush all the cloves of 1 corm of garlic and put it in a small sterilized jar. Pour pure honey over the garlic to cover and stir well. Add a bit more honey to approximately *1/2* inch above the garlic mixture and stir again. Leave it for 6 weeks to candy. Honey is a natural preservative and *the* mixture will keep indefinitely.

Take it by *the* teaspoon. One teaspoon is equivalent to 2 garlic capsules. Garlic honey is not as bad as it sounds because in 6 weeks *the* garlic taste and smell disappears, and all you can taste is honey.

Garlic Oil Capsules are readily available from health food stores. Often they can be found in regular drugstores. There is one word of advice regarding the quality of capsules, however. A gelatine capsule should begin to melt as soon as it touches *the* tongue. If you do not taste the gelatine melting, it is most likely a poor quality capsule. Some capsules mat don't dissolve easily are made with plastic and should be avoided.

I can hear you asking, "What about *the* smell?" You can rest assured. Unless you actually chew *the* garlic, whenever Garlic Oil is working on an infection, you will not smell it on *the* bream or skin. It is when you start to recover mat you begin to smell *the* garlic, and this is an indication mat it is time to cut down *the* doses as you are taking more man you need.

Part Used: The oil found in the clove

Uses: A natural antibiotic

Whenever you are advised to take a course of antibiotics, you could confidently use Garlic Oil Capsules as an alternative. Garlic Oil is pure natural sulphur and will clean up any infection anywhere in the body. It is the natural sulphur drug with no nasty side effects. Even viral infections respond to Garlic Oil. It will kill a virus without harming the host cell, a great advantage over modern antibiotics.

Since it is the oil in garlic that is desirable, when you cook with it be sure to crush the clove thoroughly to get its full goodness. For the same reason, it is best to use Garlic Oil

Capsules rather than tablets, which are made from dried garlic.

Chronic Infections

If you have been suffering any infection for a long time or have a recurring infection, you have a chronic condition. Chronic infected acne, cystitis, vaginal infections, and recurring boils are some of the classic conditions. Take 2 or 3 Garlic Oil Capsules daily, one before each meal, until the infection is gone. You will feel much better within a week. It is good insurance, however, to take it a week longer to clear up any low-grade infection.

Acute Infections

With colds, viruses, bronchitis, or any "itis," use Garlic Oil in larger doses of 3 capsules 3 times daily before meals, until it is no longer acute. Depending on the infection, this can take a few days or a week. After the acute stage, reduce the dosage to 2 or 3 capsules daily.

To explain just how powerful Garlic Oil is, in some emergency cases of blood poisoning I have prescribed up to 5 Garlic Oil Capsules each half hour for 2 days with a follow-up infection dosage. Within a few hours, the dark line that appears on the skin, moving along the bloodstream to the heart, an indication of blood poisoning, begins to disappear. In these extremely dangerous circumstances, see a practitioner immediately.

Liver Infections

If you have any liver conditions, from a mild liver infection to infectious hepatitis, Garlic Oil will cause a terrific amount of discomfort and nausea. You will need other herbs, notably Dandelion, and will need to see a practitioner.

Slippery Elm Powder

Slippery Elm Powder comes from the dried inner bark of the Slippery Elm Tree *(Ulmus fulfa)*. It is a native of Central and North American and has been a food source to several American Indian tribes.

Health food stores and herbal pharmacies can readily supply Slippery Elm Powder as well as the tablets and the dried bark. The powder, however, is the form most readily absorbed by the body and, therefore, offers the quickest relief. One 3 1/2-ounce packet of Slippery Elm Powder should meet the demand of most households for several months, unless there is a need to take it daily. It should be stored in an airtight glass jar and will keep for several years, like any properly dried herb.

When buying Slippery Elm Powder, you want 100 percent Slippery Elm. Make sure it is not adulterated. Mixed with hot water, it should form a jelly consistency. If it does not do this, the Slippery Elm bark either has not been ground finely enough, or it has been cut with something else. In either case, try another brand next time .

Part Used: The inner bark

Uses: Soother and healer of the digestive tract

Slippery Elm Powder is complete treatment for the entire digestive tract. Over acidic stomachs, nausea, ulcers, diarrhoea, constipation, bowel pockets, haemorrhoids colitis, colic, appendicitis, and even intestinal viruses all respond to Slippery Elm Powder. If your problem is anywhere in the digestive tract, Slippery Elm Powder is your answer .

One dose of Slippery Elm Powder coats the whole digestive tract, from the mouth to the rectum, with its soothing mucilage for 30 hours. It protects the lining of the digestive tract from any irritants: swallowed poisons, digestive acids, or viral infections. At the same time it coats, its rich calcium phosphates are working underneath, healing any ulcers, calming any spasms, and generally toning the digestive tract.

Dosage: One dose of Slippery Elm Powder lasts for 30 hours. No matter what the problem is, because of its last quality, the dosage is standard: 1 tablespoon of Slippery Elm Powder daily. It is best to take it at the same time each day to insure around-the-clock coverage. Though the dosage is the same for any complaint, the duration of the treatment varies.

SLIPPERY ELM SHOULD NOT BE USED FOR MORNING SICKNESS IN PREGNANCY IF YOU ARE PRONE TO MISCARRIAGE.

Slippery Elm has been known to bring on a miscarriage, but only when there is already a tendency or risk of one.

How to take Slippery Elm Powder: The craziest food combinations have been invented to help people swallow Slippery Elm Powder. As a general rule, when you need Slippery Elm you usually like the taste and don't mind the thickness, but rules always have their exceptions.

The easiest and quickest way to get it down is to mix 1 tablespoon of Slippery Elm Powder with a bit of water that has just boiled and mix it into a paste. Add a spoonful of honey for a sweet woody flavor. This way it is down the hatch with one or two swallows. If you like the flavour and don't mind the thickness, sprinkle it on your breakfast cereal or mix it with yogurt.

Though Slippery Elm Tablets are available, they take a long time to break down and do not offer the immediate relief that the powder does. Since the tablets won't start working until they reach your small intestine, your stomach will not get the benefit. So whether you like the taste or not, you will get the full benefit of Slippery Elm only from the powder.

Ulcers

Slippery Elm Powder heals both peptic and duodenal ulcers, as it works in the entire digestive tract. The ulcer is protected from the irritating digestive acids and is healed at the same time. From the first dose, the relief is immediate. In cases of an ulcer, take Slippery Elm Powder daily for 6 weeks. Even major ulcers are healed in that time.

Once the ulcer is healed and you stop taking the Slippery Elm Powder, unless you learn to live in a less frantic manner, there is nothing to insure against creating another ulcer. Changing a tense lifestyle to a more relaxed one is the only permanent ulcer treatment.

Appendicitis

Chronic or acute appendicitis is soothed very quickly with Slippery Elm Powder. The thick mucilage in Slippery Elm slides into the appendix, cleans it out, and soothes the inflammation. In the case of appendicitis, take Slippery Elm Powder daily for 6 weeks.

Gastric and Intestinal Viruses

In these cases, with their sudden and severe pain, Slippery Elm Powder is emergency treatment. Even with gastroenteritis, the pain and diarrhoea ease within seconds after taking Slippery Elm Powder. Have a tablespoon as soon as you are aware of the pain, and follow up the daily dosage for a week.

Swallowed Poisons

As soon as something harmful has been swallowed, whether poison mushrooms or lye, Slippery Elm Powder, with its heavy mucilage, will immediately protect the digestive lining from the irritant and begin to heal any damage that has been done. Though the relief is immediate, take it daily for 1 week.

Rescue Remedy

Dr. Edward Bach developed a set of flower essences and used them to balance specific emotional, mental, and spiritual states of being. They are known as Bach Flower Remedies. Rescue Remedy is one of these and is a compound of five flower essences:

Star of Bethlehem-to balance states of shock Rock Rose-to balance feelings of panic and terror
Impatiens-to balance extreme nervousness, mental stress, and tension

Cherry Plum-to balance feelings of desperation and feelings of being out of control and dangerous to oneself or others Clematis-to balance the feeling of being very far away and the "out-of-the-body" sensation

With this combination, the benefit of having Rescue Remedy in the medicine chest is obvious. Uses: To restore calm in cases of shock, panic, and extreme fear

In all cases of shock, panic, extreme fear, and the feeling of being out of the body that often accompanies these circumstances, reach for the Rescue Remedy.

It is also good for those emotional cliff-hangers, when you are feeling at the edge of the world and are ready to jump off. For any severe or prolonged nervousness, like a nervous breakdown, Rescue Remedy will ease the whole pattern and restore calm and well-being within a short time. It feels like a sigh of relief when you take it.

Whenever you find yourself crying out "Someone out there, throw me a rope!", you need some Rescue Remedy. The dosage is 10 drops for adults, 5 drops for children, directly on the tongue or in a bit of water. You may only need it once or twice, as in the case of a minor shock or pre-exam jitters. You may need a course of it, taking Rescue Remedy 3 times a day for several weeks, as in the case of a nervous breakdown. You may need to carry it around with you and take it whenever necessary, until you feel sure of yourself and your actions. In all instances, Rescue Remedy is completely safe. Take it whenever you need to be rescued.

Glossary

Alkaloid. A basic plant component containing nitrogen; for example, morphine, nicotine, quinine. When plants are used in their whole and natural forms, there is little worry of side effects, as the plants are balanced and kept in check by the other substances in the plant.

Antibiotic. A substance that prohibits the growth of bacterial infection. Herbs with an antibiotic action, like garlic, do not harm helpful bacteria.

Antiseptic. A remedy that destroys bacterial infection. Herbs with an antiseptic action inhibit the growth of harmful bacteria only.

Antispasmodic. A remedy that prevents and relieves muscular spasms.

Expectorant. A remedy that promotes coughing and, therefore, the release of phlegm from the throat and lungs.

Emollient. A remedy that soothes and softens externally.

Fungicide. A remedy that destroys fungus.

Glycoside. A basic plant compound containing a simple sugar. Herbs high in glycoside content usually have a laxative effect and are blood cleansing in their action.

Liniment. An oily liquid preparation for external use. It is applied by massage into the skin and muscles.

Ointment. A smooth, greasy preparation for the external use of healing the skin. It is applied on dressings or by rubbing into the skin.

Phytosteroids. A plant component containing hormones and vitamins in a natural balance.

Poultice. A soft mass spread on a dressing and applied to a sore or inflamed area of the body.

Septic. The putrid, infected, festering state of a wound.

Sedative. A remedy that has a soothing and calming action on the nervous system.

Soporific. A remedy that induces sleep.

Styptic. A remedy that stops bleeding.

Sources of Herbs and Herb Products

All of the products listed in this book are readily available, though you may have to look beyond the familiar drug store. Health food stores, herbal pharmacies, and food co-ops are usually the best sources of herbal products. Even if there is no such store nearby, there are many mail-order businesses that carry these products.

www.ingramcontent.com/pod-product-compliance
Lightning Source LLC
Chambersburg PA
CBHW071004290526
45795CB00005B/1769